The Immunocytes and transplantation

Donate an organ to save a life

Author – Editor: Juan Carlos Aldave

Jr. Domingo Cueto 371, Dpto. 301, Lince

Lima – Perú

Phone: (+51) 948-323-720

jucapul_84@hotmail.com

First Edition: November 2015

ISBN: 978-1519481207

November 2015

Since birth we are exposed to dangerous microbes than put our life at risk. So, we need several cells and molecules capable of defending our body. We will call "immune system" to our body defenses, and "immunocytes" to the immune cells that protect us.

Some people have a vital organ or tissue severely damaged. They need a transplant to continue living. The immunocytes are very strong and powerful to attack bad microbes. However, they must tolerate foreign molecules in the transplanted graft.

In this little book we will see the main risks and complications of organ and tissue transplantation.

Index

Do you know that transplants save lives?

Treg

Chapter 1:
The immunocytes defend us

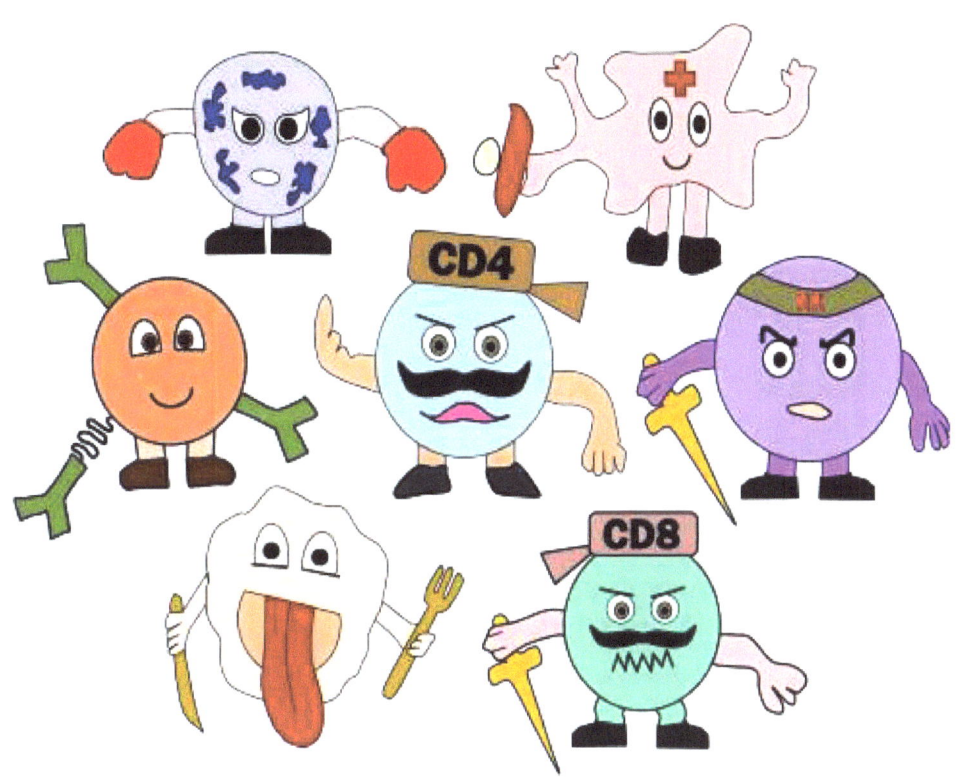

The main role of our immunocytes is to defend us from the dangerous microbes and cancerous cells that threaten our life. For example, the TH1 battalion destroys the lethal *Mycobacterium tuberculosis*, the TH17 battalion eliminates the fungus *Candida albicans*, and the anti-cancer army kills malignant cells.

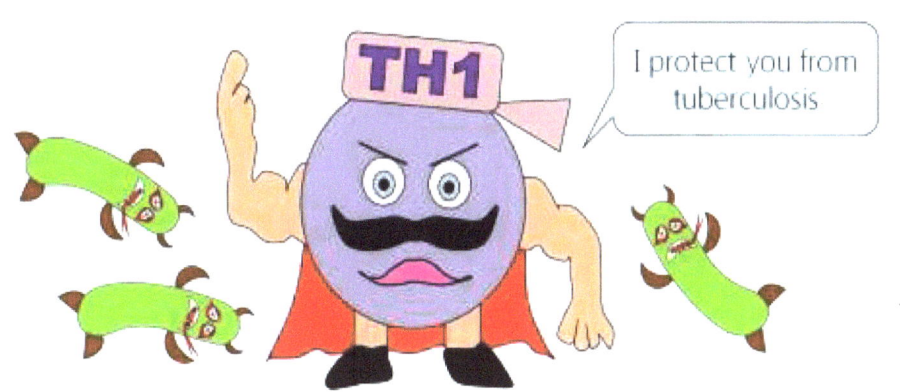

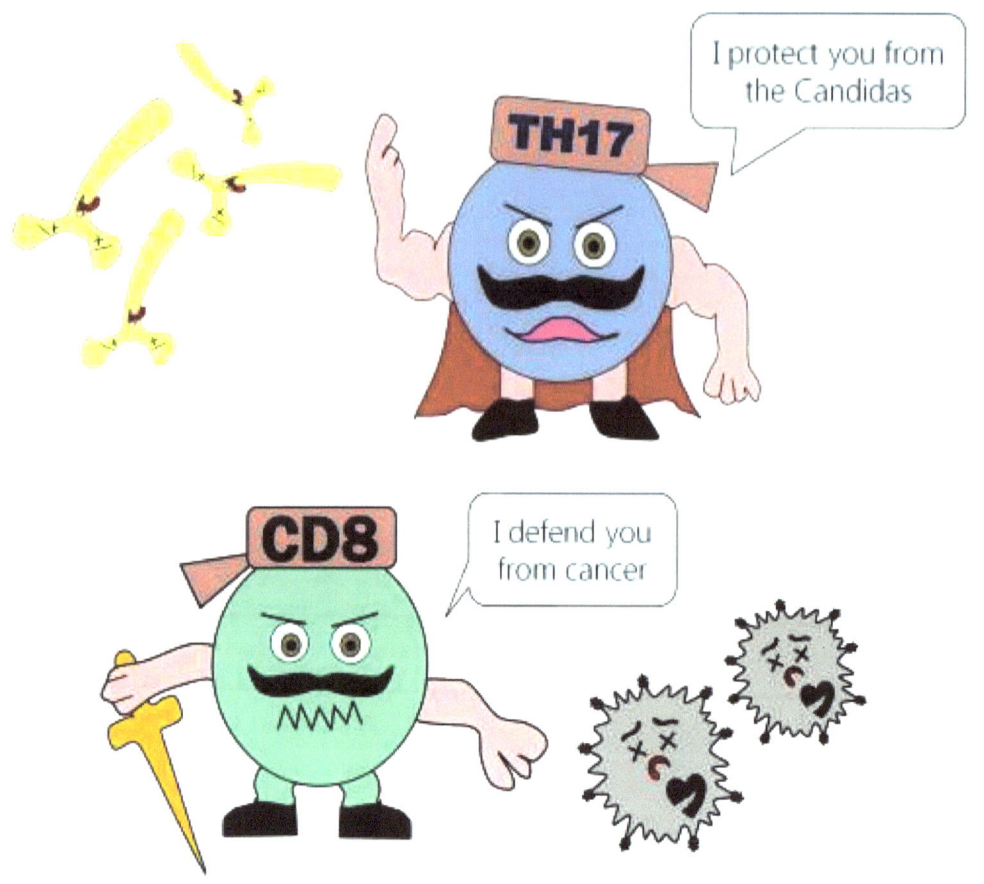

Our immunocytes are very powerful. They activate quickly after detecting dangerous foreign molecules in our body to remove them and thus preserve life.

However, there are molecules that, despite being foreign, are beneficial to the organism. Therefore, these molecules must be tolerated by the immune system. For example, the molecules in an organ or tissue that is transplanted from another subject. The processes of immune tolerance are favored by the T regulatory cell.

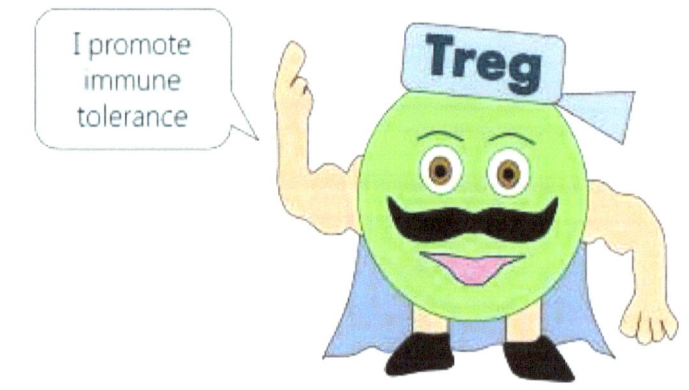

Chapter 2:
When an organ or tissue fails

Our body is formed by several organ and tissues that function coordinately to generate life. For example:

- The brain is the source and receptor of nerve impulses that allow us to move, think and feel.

- Our heart pumps blood carrying oxygen and nutrients to other organs. Lungs oxygenate the blood.

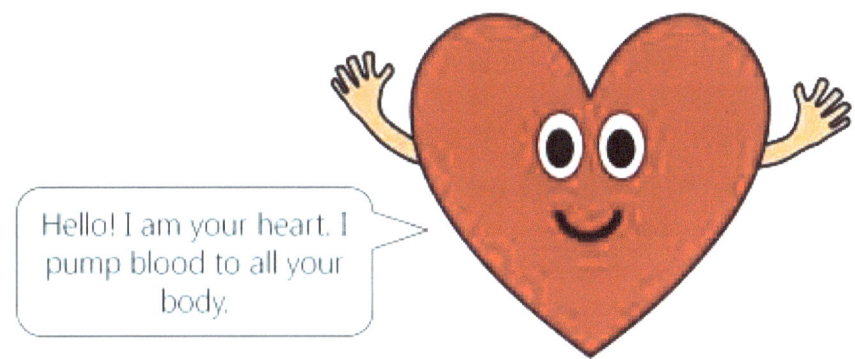

- Our liver and kidneys remove toxic substances from the body.

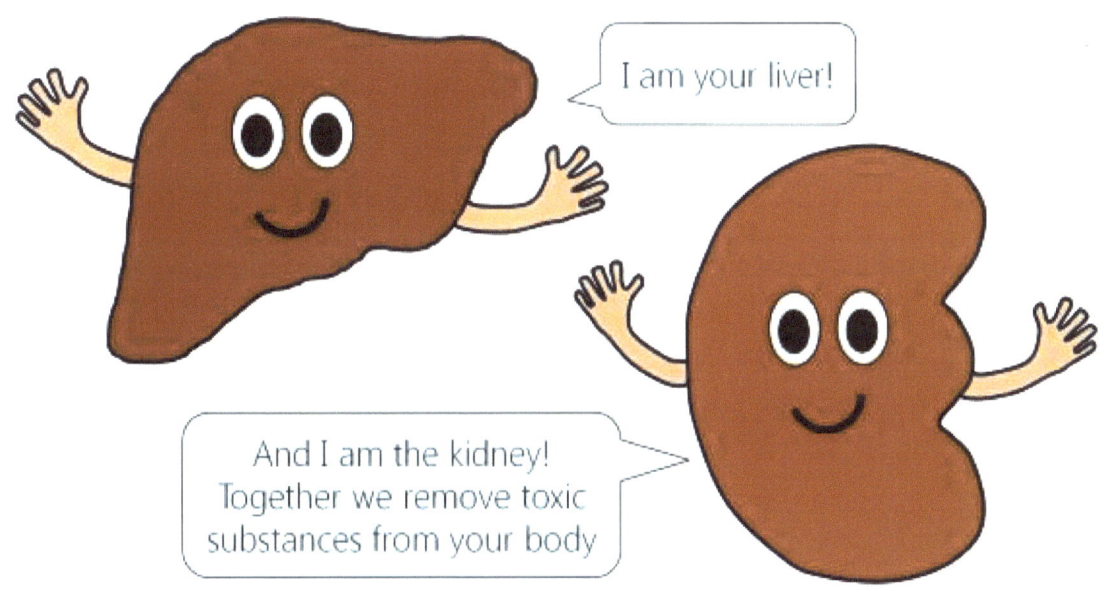

- The stomach and intestines let us feed and grow.

- Bone marrow contains millions of hematopoietic stem cells, which function as the factory of blood cells (red blood cells, leukocytes or immunocytes, and platelets).

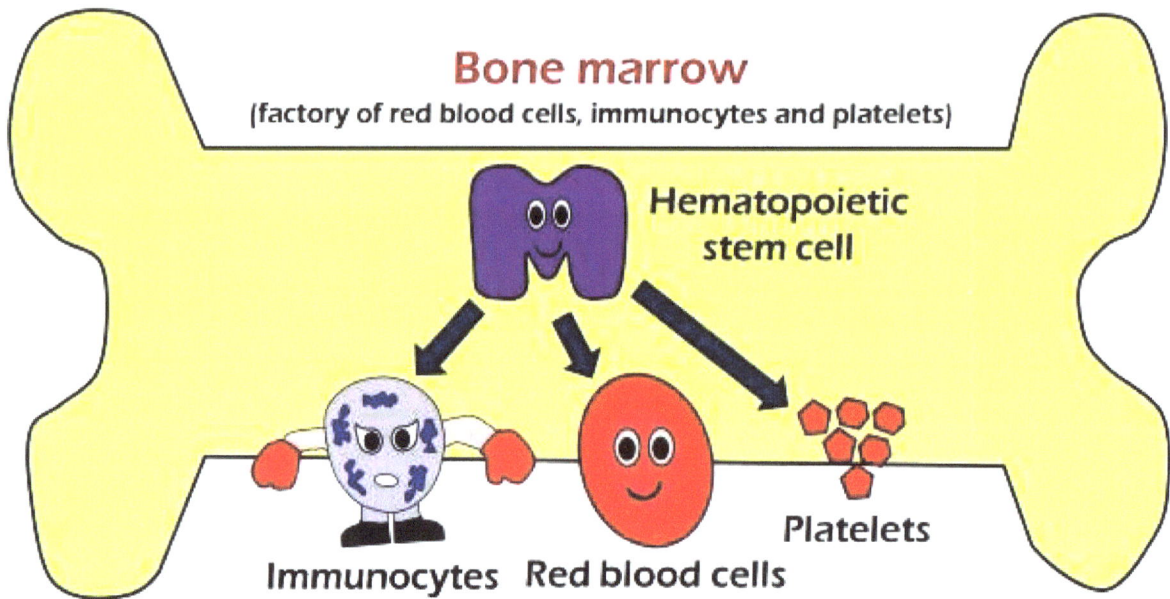

Unfortunately, certain diseases cause a severe damage to vital organs and tissues, directly jeopardizing the patient's life. For instance:

- Arterial hypertension and coronary disease damage heart cells and produce congestive heart failure.

- Cigarette smoke generates chronic lung damage.

- Excessive alcohol consumption and certain hepatitis viruses destroy liver cells and cause cirrhosis.

- Diabetes mellitus and arterial hypertension damage kidney cells, causing chronic renal disease.

- Some genetic abnormalities induce a permanent injury in the bone marrow, affecting the normal production of blood cells.

Chapter 3: The process of organ and tissue transplantation

There are people who have a vital organ or tissue severely damaged. To continue living or improve quality of life, these patients are candidates to receive an 'allogeneic transplant', that is, a healthy organ or tissue coming from another subject. For example:

- Patients with severe heart failure need a heart transplant.

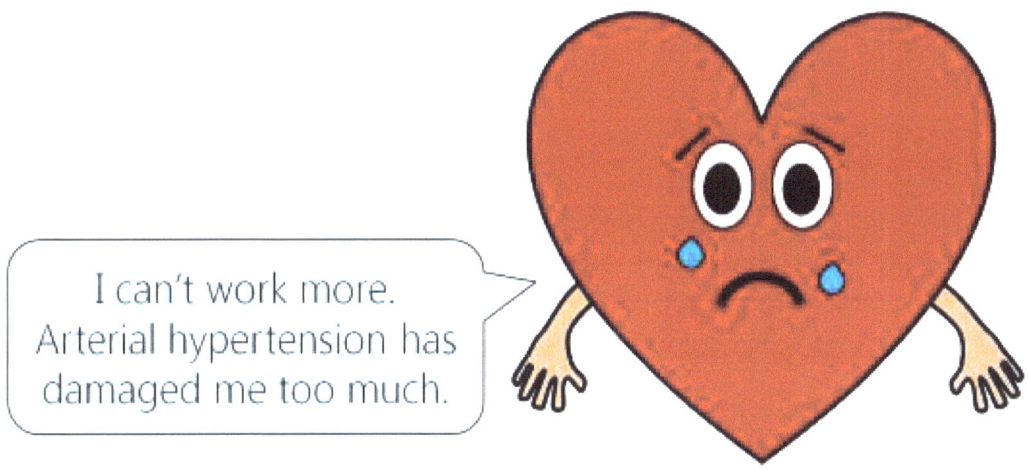

I can't work more. Arterial hypertension has damaged me too much.

- Subjects with severe chronic lung disease require new healthy lungs.

- Liver transplantation can save the life of patients with advanced cirrhosis.

- People with end-stage renal disease can be cured with a kidney transplant.

- Children with severe diseases affecting the bone marrow need healthy hematopoietic stem cells (bone marrow transplantation).

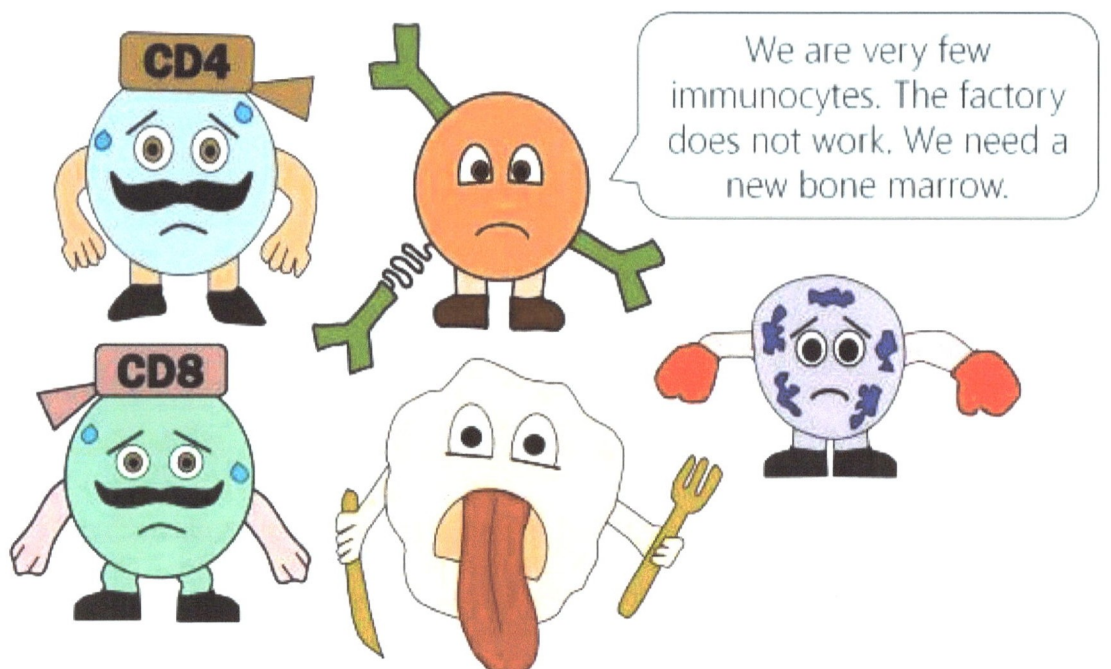

Organ or tissue transplantation is often complex and expensive. To perform a successful transplant it is necessary:

- A suitable and responsible patient (recipient).

- A qualified donor, compatible with the recipient. Some transplants are done from a living donor, others from a deceased donor.

- A supportive family, with faith and trust.

- Trained health personnel.

- Appropriate infrastructure and equipment.

- Permanent availability of the required medicines.

- Sufficient financial and administrative resources.

The transplant process has several risks, especially for the recipient. Therefore, it is essential to prevent, detect and treat complications in time.

Chapter 4:
The risks of transplantation

The process of organ and tissue transplantation may present some difficulties. In the following picture you can see common transplant complications.

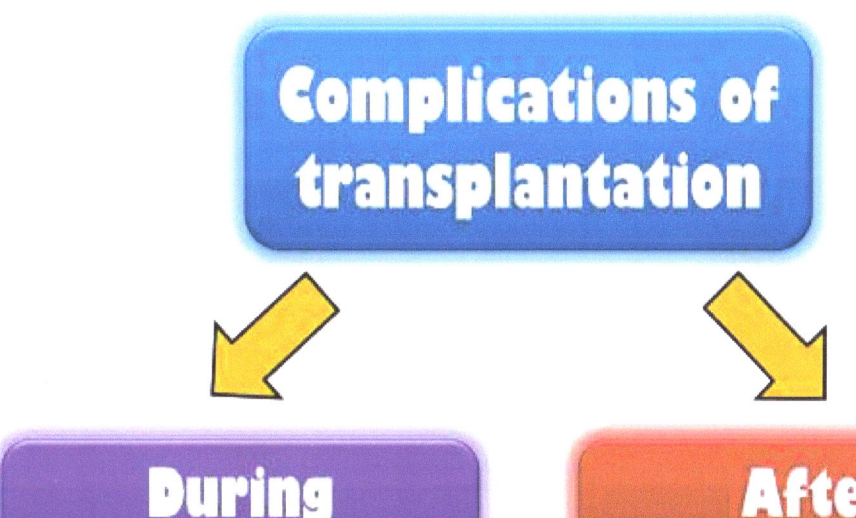

Complications of transplantation

During transplantation
- **Blood loss during surgery (bone marrow transplantation does not require major surgery)**
- **Allergic reactions**
- **Other surgical complications**

After transplantation
- **Infections**
- **Incompatibility between donor and recipient**
- **Adverse effects of medications**
- **Other postoperative complications**

Complications that occur during and after the transplant may result in the loss of the graft, jeopardizing the patient's life and significantly increasing proceedings costs.

Therefore, it is essential to prevent such complications. For instance:

- During surgery it is necessary to have some blood units compatible with the recipient in case of excessive blood loss. In addition, the patient must enter the operating room with an acceptable level of hemoglobin. Surgery should be as perfect as possible; surgeon's experience is essential.

- Before transplantation surgery the anesthesiology physician should perform a risk assessment, including patient's allergy history.

- It is essential to know the adverse effects of the medicines that will be used, and to warn the patient, in order to detect them early.

In the next two chapters I will explain you some medical recommendations to reduce the risk of infections and graft rejection.

Please answer the following questions:

1. Write two complications that can occur during transplantation:

   _____

   _____

2. List 3 possible complications after transplantation:

   _____

   _____

   _____

Chapter 5:
Preventing graft rejection

Several molecules in the transplanted organ or tissue can be recognized as foreign by the immune system of the recipient. When this occurs, the recipient's immunocytes are able to attack and destroy the graft. This complication is known as 'graft rejection'.

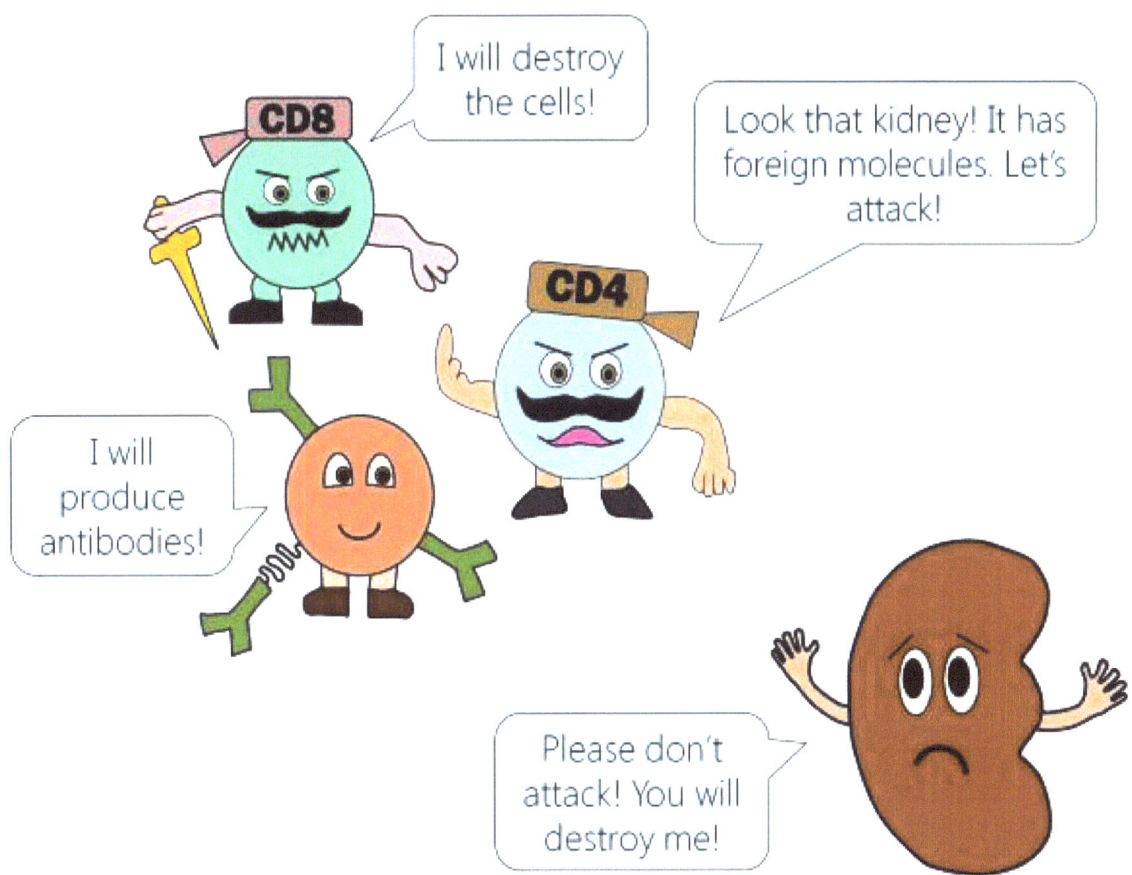

To prevent graft rejection it is necessary to inhibit the recipient's immune system. The medicines that accomplish this purpose are called 'immunosuppressive drugs', such as corticosteroids (eg. prednisone, methylprednisolone, dexamethasone), cyclosporine, tacrolimus, everolimus, mycophenolate, azathioprine and some monoclonal antibodies (eg. Daclizumab, Basiliximab).

Unfortunately, immunosuppressive drugs cause two common complications:

- Adverse reactions, which vary according to the required drugs and individual patient characteristics.

- Immunodeficiency, that is, a reduction in the power of the immunocytes. This state predisposes the patient to the attack by several life-threatening microbes.

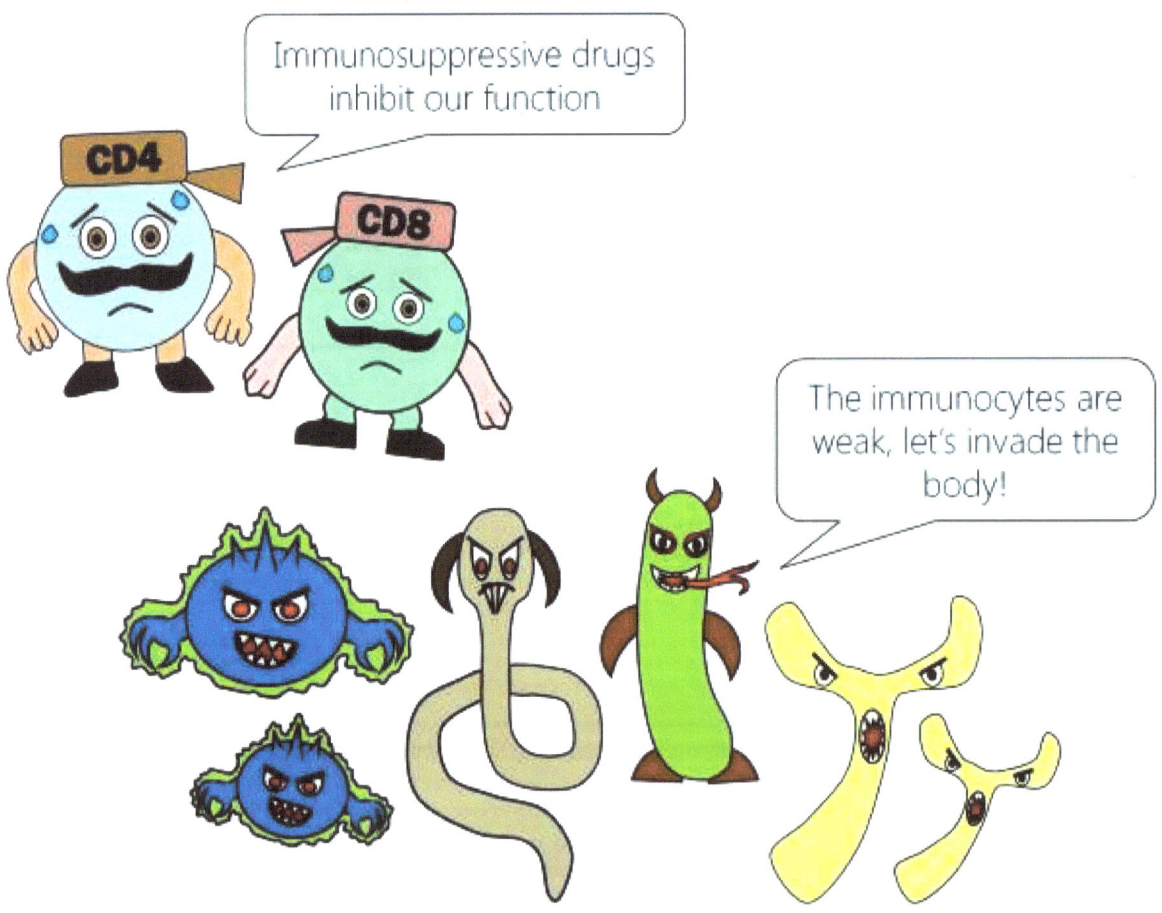

Let's continue to chapter number six, where we will see how to reduce the risk of infections associated with the use of immunosuppressive drugs.

Chapter 6:
Preventing infections

After receiving a transplant, patients are medicated with immunosuppressive drugs to prevent graft rejection. However, the state of immunodeficiency caused by such drugs predispose to several infections.

Let's understand some recommendations to prevent the invasion by potentially lethal microbes:

- Transplanted patients often require antimicrobial drugs prophylactically. For example: cotrimoxazole to prevent lung infection by *Pneumocystis jiroveci*, nystatin to prevent the growth of *Candida albicans*, isoniazid to stop the reproduction of *Mycobacterium tuberculosis*, and ganciclovir to block the attack of cytomegalovirus.

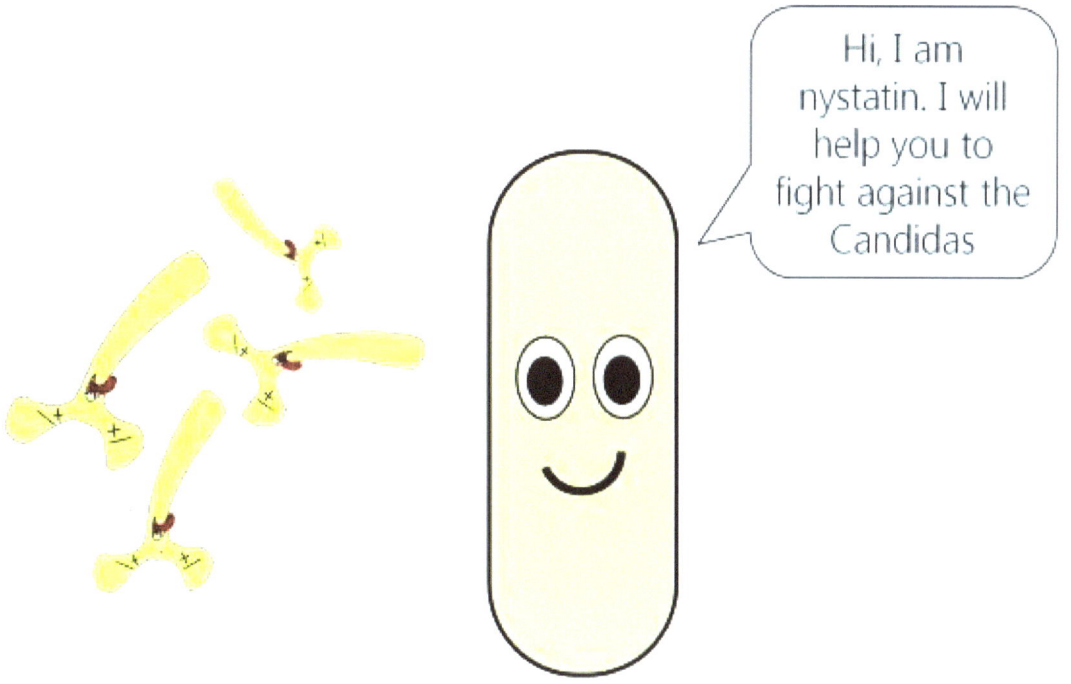

Hi, I am nystatin. I will help you to fight against the Candidas

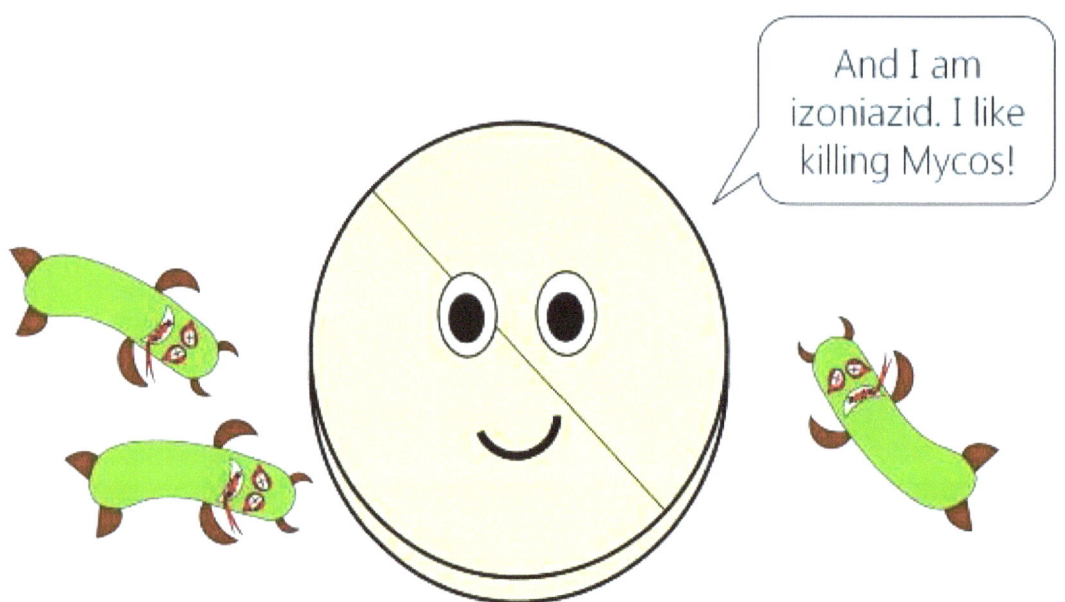

- It is very important to detect infections promptly. So, patients must be alert. It is the patient's responsibility to consult his/her physician at the minimal sign of infection or any unexplained discomfort.

- The patient and his/her family should actively collaborate with the recommendations of isolation during the period of immunosuppression. For example: use protective masks properly, wash hands frequently, avoid contact to individuals with active infections, eat uncontaminated food, maintain good hygiene at home, etc.

- It is essential to optimize the medical management of comorbidities (eg. diabetes mellitus, hypertension) and maintain an adequate nutritional status.

Transplant success increases substantially if we fulfill the recommendations to reduce the risk of infections and graft rejection.

Chapter 7:
Saving lives with transplantation

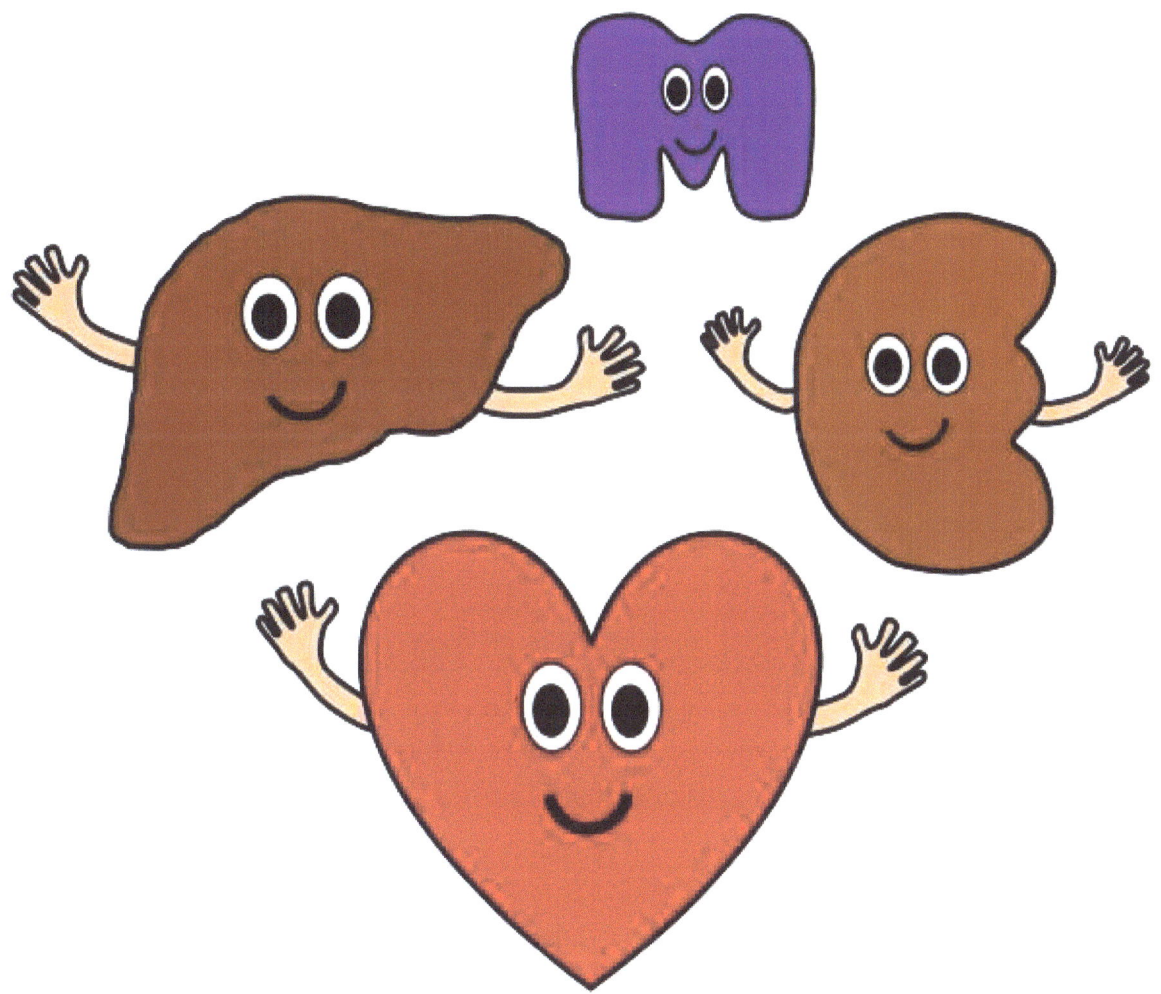

Millions of people worldwide still live because they got a transplant opportunely. However, many more people die without receiving a transplant in time. Moreover, a significant percentage of transplants fail because graft rejection, infections or surgical complications.

Can we optimize the transplant process?

In the previous chapters we learned some recommendations to reduce the risk of transplant-associated complications.

It is important to enhance immune tolerance towards the transplanted organ or tissue. A great challenge, in constant research, is generating T regulatory lymphocytes specific to foreign molecules in the graft.

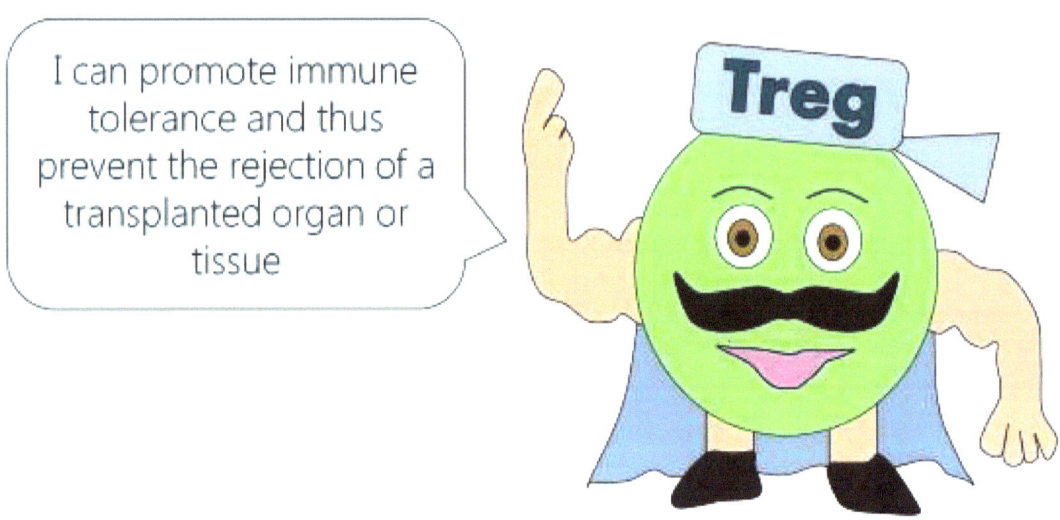

I can promote immune tolerance and thus prevent the rejection of a transplanted organ or tissue

Why there are not enough transplants?

Lack of donors is a major constraint to perform more transplants. Many people are afraid to donate an organ, even after death. This fear is often unfounded.

Every individual must understand that transplants are essential procedures to prolong the life of patients with a severely damaged organ or tissue.

There are many people who need a healthy organ or tissue to continue living.
Donate an organ! Save a life!

In this little book we learned about the importance of transplantation to give life to patients with a severely damaged organ or tissue.

Do not miss the following book, where we will understand the lethal attack of human immunodeficiency virus to our immunocytes.

Juan Carlos Aldave, MD
Allergy and Clinical Immunology

Contributors:

- Dr. Juan Félix Aldave Pita
- Bertha Alicia Becerra Sánchez

"For God so loved the world that he gave his one and only Son, that whoever believes in him shall not perish but have eternal life". John 3:16

10 Warning Signs
of Primary Immunodeficiency

Primary Immunodeficiency (PI) causes children and adults to have infections that come back frequently or are unusually hard to cure. 1:500 persons are affected by one of the known Primary Immunodeficiencies. **If you or someone you know is affected by two or more of the following Warning Signs, speak to a physician about the possible presence of an underlying Primary Immunodeficiency.**

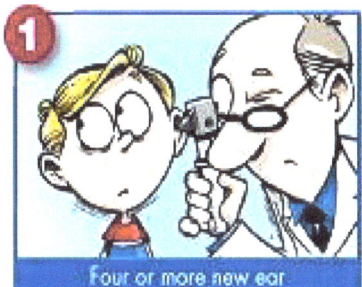
1 Four or more new ear infections within one year.

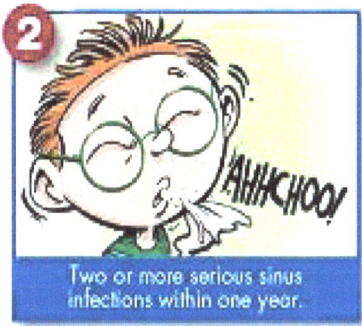
2 Two or more serious sinus infections within one year.

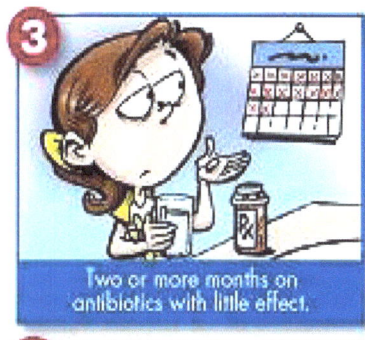
3 Two or more months on antibiotics with little effect.

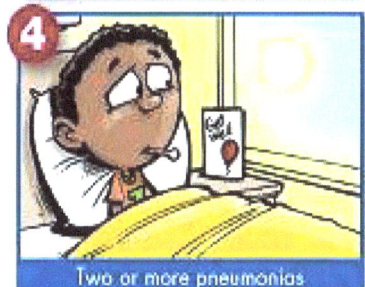
4 Two or more pneumonias within one year.

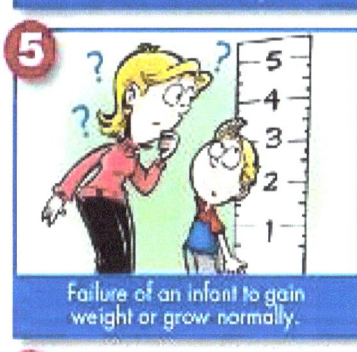
5 Failure of an infant to gain weight or grow normally.

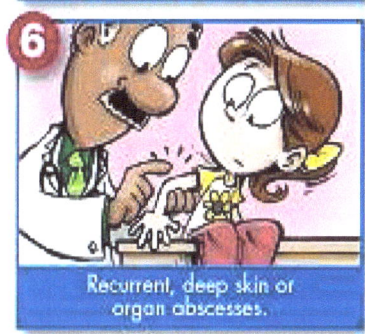
6 Recurrent, deep skin or organ abscesses.

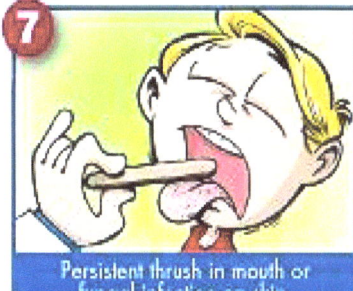
7 Persistent thrush in mouth or fungal infection on skin.

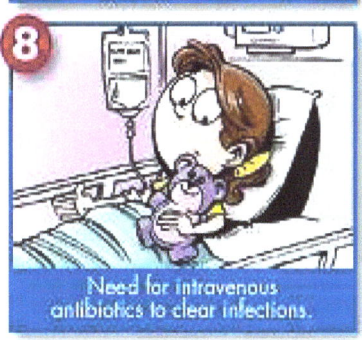
8 Need for intravenous antibiotics to clear infections.

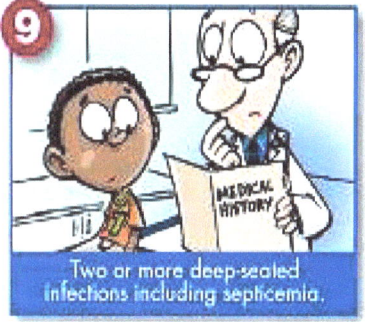
9 Two or more deep-seated infections including septicemia.

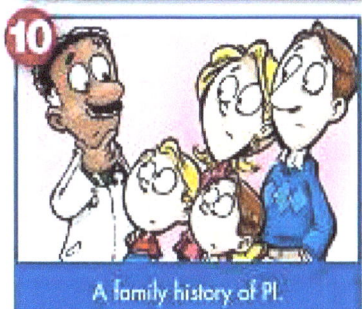
10 A family history of PI.

"These warning signs were developed by the Jeffrey Modell Foundation Medical Advisory Board. Consultation with Primary Immunodeficiency experts is strongly suggested. ©2013 Jeffrey Modell Foundation"

www.INFO4PI.org

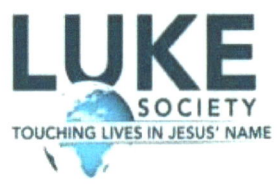

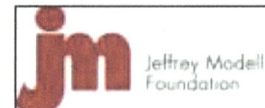

Series: Funny Immunology to Save Lives

(Editions in English and Spanish)

Book 1:   The Immunocytes
Book 2:   The TH17 army against Candida
Book 3:   The TH1 army against Mycobacteria
Book 4:   The TH2 army against worms
Book 5:   The battle against Pneumococcus
Book 6:   The immunocytes against cancer
Book 7:   T regs: controlling the immune army
Book 8:   When the Immunocytes get sick...
Book 9:   When the Immunocytes go crazy...
Book 10:   The Immunocytes and transplantation
Book 11:   The armor of the Immunocyte Felix

Contact the Author:
Jirón Domingo Cueto 371, Of. 301, Lince, LIMA 14
Lima, Peru
Phones: +51 948-323-720
          +51 988-689-472
jucapul_84@hotmail.com
funny.immunology@gmail.com
www.alergomed.org/immunocytes

www.ingramcontent.com/pod-product-compliance
Lightning Source LLC
Chambersburg PA
CBHW041320180526
45172CB00004B/1167